Compassionate
Caring for the Sick and Dying

Sara Arline Thrash

D0555932

TWENTY-THIRD PUBLICATIONS
BAYARD Mystic, CT 06355

Acknowledgments

Gratitude is the hallmark of a caring heart, and my gratitude overflows to the following at Tampa General Hospital:

Dan McRight, Clinical Pastoral Education Director, whose office door was always wide enough for crash landings.

Glennys Ulschack, Staff Chaplain, whose earthy vitamins of wisdom and hilarious joy cooled my head, warmed my heart, and nourished my soul.

Cellion Altene, Clinical Pastoral Supervisor, who walked by my side along the path.

My patients, who allowed me to sit by their hearth fires and hear their stories.

And to Neil Kluepfel, Publisher of Twenty-Third Publications, who has a vision for caregiving, and Deborah McCann, Editorial Consultant to Twenty-Third Publications, whose keen organization and sequencing skills brought focus to the vision of caregiving.

Except where indicated in the text, the Scripture passages contained herein are from the *New Revised Standard Version of the Bible,* copyright © 1989, by the Division of Christian Education of the National Council of Churches of Christ in the U.S.A. All rights reserved.

Twenty-Third Publications/Bayard
185 Willow Street
P.O. Box 180
Mystic, CT 06355
(860) 536-2611
(800) 321-0411

ISBN:1-58595-004-1
Library of Congress Catalog Card Number: 99-75664
Printed in the U.S.A.

"Being called by God to minister as a chaplain requires a heart of compassion as big as the heart God gave Sara Thrash. This book will enrich peoples' lives beyond measure."

Chaplain Robert M. Brooks, Jr.
The Baptist Home, Ozark, MO

"This gentle, yet mighty book is about people coming together, stretching far beyond the limits of roles and diagnoses where people, not roles or symptoms, are bonded by the binding love of God."

Rev. Dr. Richard B. Gilbert
Executive Director, The World Pastoral Care Center

"The next time I am hospitalized—I hope God sends Sara Thrash or a hospital chaplain who has read this important book."

Harold Ivan Smith
Author, *A Decembered Grief: Living with Loss When Others Are Celebrating*

"I highly recommend this book for all who are interested in pastoral care. It shows clearly the priesthood of all believers and should be equally valuable to ministers and lay people."

Dan A. McRight
Baptist Health System of South Florida

"This book title expresses Arline Thrash's own attitude of compassion and caring. It should prove meaningful to many readers."

Paul D. Brewer
Carson-Newman College, Jefferson City, TN

"Dr. Sara Thrash is a gifted writer who knows what it means to be called by God and she carries out that calling with a genuine servant-like spirit and commitment."

Maurice G. Cook, PhD
Professor Emeritus, North Carolina State University

"Sara Thrash shares deep insights of human emotions and frailties, gleaned from her own life and those of her patients."

Aubrey Beauchamp RN
USA Coordinator Hospital, Christian Fellowship International

"This will be a book which I not only highly recommend, but will use in my practice and seminars."

Chip Whitman, M.A., Director, Grief Care
San Juan Capistrano, CA

"With wisdom and insight, Sara Thrash encourages patients to own their feelings, rather than fight or suppress them. This is a sanity saver, and helps people to understand themselves better, and thus to deal better with the situation."

Pat Egan Dexter, O.P.L.
Author, *Coping as Caregivers*

"Clergy in congregations, chaplains, pastoral counselors, nurses and physicians, take note: this book is for you."

Rev. Glennys Ulschak
Lawrence & Memorial Hospital, New London, CT

"This book should be required reading for ALL medical doctors and part of a minister's essential handbook before ordination."

Betty Malz
Author, *My Glimpse of Eternity, Heaven: A Bright and Glorious Place*

"Sara Thrash, in her book *Compassionate Caring for the Sick and Dying*, explores death and dying in a magnificent way, and she leaves the reader well prepared for a future of inescapable events that are a part of life."

Carl Malz
Writer/Minister, Crystal Beach, FL

For Laura Cate and Andrew Mark Thrash
Precious grandtwins who have blessed me with
seven years of caregiving
and
For Phillip Douglas Thrash
Beloved new caregiver

"Let the little children come to me,
do not stop them;
for it is to such as these
that the kingdom of God belongs."
Mark 10:14

Contents

Introduction 1

Part I—Our Role as Caregivers
(what we need to know or do)

Why Do Patients Fear Death? 4
Struggling with a Patient's Death 7
Walking with Grieving Families 11
Assisting Families in Saying their Good-byes 16
Giving Family Members Permission to Cry 20
Becoming Kingdom Scarecrows 24
Listening with Our Hearts 27

Part II—Understanding Our Patients
(what they're telling us in their words and by their actions)

Addressing the Concerns of Children Facing Death 32
Why? 37
Allowing Patients to "Own" their Feelings 41
Coping with Attention-Seeking Patients 47

Part III—Learning and Growing Together
(sharing feelings, spirituality, concerns)

Symbols of Faith 52
Despair 54
Laughter 58
Thanking God in All Circumstances 62
A Praying Heart 65

For Further Reading 70

Introduction

More people pass through the hospitals of the world in a given year than through its churches. Hospitals can be fearful places in which both patients and their families experience uncertainty, sadness, discordance, helplessness, and loneliness. When we volunteer to visit with the sick, we have a God-given opportunity to touch the lives of those who are weary and broken in spirit with an unhurried presence and a listening, caring heart.

When a family member requires hospitalization, it upsets the equilibrium of the entire family. Family members often need as much nurturing and emotional support as the patient does.

Patients are often denied the wish to speak realistically of death by well-meaning family members, and family members are met with a "Do Not Disturb" sign when trying to approach the subject with their loved ones. Survivor's guilt, particularly in auto accidents or swift disease and death, takes a heavy toll when family members continue to dwell on why they were spared and their loved ones taken.

Life and death medical decisions—placing a loved one on life-support, dialysis, or subjecting the member to a surgical procedure—place extreme pressure on the family even when the loved one has registered a decision prior to hospitalization. Accepting the reality of the situation and the impossibility of cure is extremely difficult. Acknowledging—or denying—the hopelessness of the situation overwhelms family members as they struggle with this heavy burden. Such a decision often divides and tears the family apart. Through all this maze, the caregiver must walk with eyes, ears, heart, and spirit open.

This book is written to support, affirm, encourage, and nurture the myriad volunteer caregivers who visit hospitals, convalescent and nursing homes, life-care facilities, and home settings in thousands of parishes and communities. My prayer is that it will also touch those professionally and pastorally involved with the care of the sick. By taking the time to understand our role as caregivers, to address the problems and concerns of those we comfort, and to work on our own healthy spirituality so that we can share it with others, we will become beacons of light in the darkness of fear and dread, and be God's true representatives to those we visit.

Our Role as Caregivers

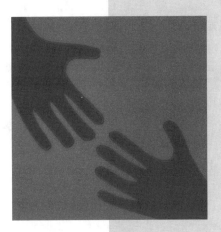

What we need to know or do

Why Do Patients Fear Death?

"Dear God, What is it like when you die? Nobody will tell me. I just want to know. I don't want to do it. Your friend, Mike."

That young boy's question, from Stuart Hample and Eric Marshall's book *Children's Letters to God*, is ageless. What is death like? Alas, we don't want to talk about this taboo subject, yet the fear of death remains the greatest fear of humankind because it is the Great Unknown. As one teenager put it, "Lazarus hasn't appeared at Tampa General to walk us through death."

We are guilty of complicating the subject of death even further by the very language we use to describe it. We deny death: "He passed away. She is asleep. They've gone home. He left us. She's gone on a long trip." We camouflage death, conceal it cosmetically, and even use artificial turf to mask the wound in the earth where the casket will be placed. We try to protect our children from its reality and finality. Is it any wonder patients fear death with all its mystery?

My patients tell me they don't fear death nearly as much as the process of dying—how they will die. I share their feelings. What if dying takes weeks or months of suffering, of dying inch by inch? I don't want to be a burden to my loved ones, to be of no help to anyone, to be of no earthly use! I hope I go quickly with no physical care required and no draining of my family's finances.

Some of my patients, especially those with little or no belief in the hereafter, express their fear of being forgotten, of fading away to obscurity, to limbo, to the end of their existence, unremembered by their grandchildren or other extended family members: "Death is so final."

A few patients expressed grief over physical rejection and disdain of their horrible appearance. "My sons come to the hospital as infrequently as possible. They can't stand to see me in this pitiful condition, to even touch me. So they don't come, and that isolates me even more and makes me feel unclean and unworthy of their time and attention."

Female patients express their great fear of separation more than male patients do. "My family still needs me. How can I leave my children and grandchildren? Will we know each other in heaven? Will we recognize our loved ones?"

More males than females, however, speak of leaving work unfinished, of leaving goals they've set unreached. Dreams, hopes, aspirations, and unrealized potential weigh more heavily upon them. Robert Frost's "I have miles to go before I sleep" reflects their mindsets. Four of my male patients, however, have confided to me, "Chaplain, if I had to do it all over again, I would spend far less time at the office or with my business and far more time with my wife and children. Why do you have to be flat on your back before you finally figure out what the most important things are in your life?"

Professional and volunteer caregivers can help patients to face their fears with honesty by allowing patients to ventilate concerns and ask questions instead of concealing them. Just being there for a patient nearing death is such comfort. Don't fear silences. Your very presence is one of the answers to the question, "Does God really care?" You don't have to defend God. Be very attentive to body language. Often a patient will try to grasp your hand, a signal that he or she wants to tell you something. It is of the utmost importance at times like this simply to be at peace with God and yourself. Patients will be able to pick up on your agitation or discomfort. Your physical touch gently conveys to the patient, "I am here for you."

Never forget you are God's earthly representative to your

patient. A dear old dying saint in India asked our senior chaplain to come and sit with her in her last hour and read Psalm 63:

O God, you are my God, I seek you,
my soul thirsts for you;
my flesh faints for you,
as in a dry and weary land where there is no water.
So I have looked upon you in the sanctuary,
beholding your power and glory.
Because your steadfast love is better than life,
my lips will praise you.
So I will bless you as long as I live.

Sister Grace, tears washing down her face as she smiled at us, reported when she read the line, "Your love is better than life itself," the patient broke into the most beautiful smile, and she drew her last breath as Sister Grace read, "So I will bless you as long as I live."

Prayer

"I think of you on my bed, and meditate on you in the watches of the night; for you have been my help, and in the shadow of your wings I sing for joy. My soul clings to you; your right hand upholds me."
(Psalm 63:6–8)

Abba Father,
Our patient did not get to these verses, Lord. She entered your presence blessing you with all her life. What a testimony of faith! Jesus, remind us every time we walk into a hospital room we are there as your representative. Let everything we say or do reflect your unconditional love for this patient. You are the Big Physician whose bedside manner has never been improved! Accept my limitations and use me for your glory.

Struggling with a Patient's Death

As a chaplain I experience a kaleidoscope of emotions when one of my patients dies. Does God really care about our grief, our pain, our fragility, our vulnerability? That question assaults me briefly when I stand with grieving parents and cry out inaudibly, "I believe; help my unbelief!" (Mark 9:24). Tears of sadness engulf me as I share the agony of parents struggling with their broken dreams and breached expectations. On the other hand, tears of relief and gratitude soar upward at the homegoing of a suffering patient who has lived long and well.

My greatest struggle with a patient's death ended in a glorious symphony of God's love and peace, played in my presence by the patient's parents.

Only thirty-two, he awaited a heart transplant when a donor could be found. Beloved by his parents from Sarasota, he was the recipient of prayers from his family, church, city, and concerned ones throughout the nation. Seldom have I seen a family so encircled by love and faith. Alas, he developed pneumonia, and as it worsened his name was removed from the recipient list. He was now comatose in Cardiac Intensive Care with his life hanging by a very slim thread.

His parents, sustained by their faith in God and the presence of friends, slipped in and out of his room several times each day. To see the love in their eyes as they watched over this son was heart-wrenching. I have three sons and I kept watch over two of them in their very young years as they slipped to eternity's edge and then returned to us.

One morning the parents came in with a small vial of oil and asked me to go with them to his bedside and anoint him as we prayed the Prayer for the Sick as recorded in James

5:14–15. I was honored to do so and we prayed, "Are any among you sick? They should call for the elders of the church and have them pray over them, anointing them with oil in the name of the Lord. The prayer of faith will save the sick, and the Lord will raise them up; and anyone who has committed sins will be forgiven."

When I came in early the next morning a nurse told me my patient had died in the night. When death comes, it takes far more than the life of a patient. Never do we parents expect to outlive our children. When we lose our parents, we lose a part of our past. But when our children die before we do, they take the future with them.

"O Jesus, what will I say to them? What will I say? They had more faith when I anointed their son than I had! I'm sorry I lacked their faith. What will I say?"

I need not have worried or agonized. Those parents encircled me with their arms and held me tightly as I began to speak and then fell apart. "Sara, God who was God two weeks ago when our son was alive and awaiting a transplant is still God today! We prayed for healing and God has given our son the ultimate healing. He has raised him up. Blessed be the name of the Lord." I still have the tiny vial with a few drops of oil on my bedroom dresser to remind me that the God of yesterday is the God of today, sufficient for every need or heart scald we experience.

Four years later in India, I sat by the bedside of a beloved retired pastor in the last stages of cancer, his frail body beset by pain that no drug could lessen for more than an hour. Each day as I visited in his room, his eyes told me so much that he could not say in the presence of his family. He was returned to the Intensive Care Unit, where he summoned me late one afternoon. Motioning me to bend over his face, he removed the oxygen mask. As I held his weather-beaten hand in mine, a tear dropped on his cheek.

"Chaplain, my old earthly tent is falling down and I want nothing more than to see the face of my Savior. My family keeps clinging to me and crying not to leave them. Try again to tell them I'm ready to go. Please help them to let me go."

At midnight the family frantically summoned me from the dorm to come to the chapel. I slipped in to see my patient first. Celestial peace had settled into his being. "I'm going," he whispered.

I sat in the chapel with the family for half an hour. Looking straight at them, I said very quietly, "Your husband and father is slipping into eternity. Please don't hold him back any longer. He asked you to release him so he could see the face of Jesus this very night."

Word of his death came to me the next morning at chaplains' meeting. Tears of gratitude to God and joy for my patient coursed down my face.

The beloved apostle, John, records Jesus' words to Mary Magdalene after his resurrection. "Do not hold on to me…go to my brothers and say to them, 'I am ascending to my Father and your Father, to my God and your God'" (John 20:16–17).

How I long to tell families, "Do not hold on to your loved one who is longing to see the face of the Savior. Rather, go and tell others that your beloved one has returned to his Father and your Father, to my God and your God!"

Caregivers, be aware that you will also experience an ambivalent kaleidoscope of emotions as you minister to the dying. Ask for God's discernment when sorting out your feelings. "Trust in the Lord with all your heart and do not rely on your own insight" (Proverbs 3:5). You who have spent many hours with a patient can influence family members to "let go" by giving them honest feedback from the patient and redemptively listening to them as they pour out their feelings and express their concerns. If you've had a personal experience in "letting go," this may be an appropriate time to share it in love.

Prayer

*"May those who sow in tears reap with shouts of joy. Those
who go out weeping, bearing the seed for sowing, shall
come home with shouts of joy, carrying their sheaves"
(Psalm 126:5–6)*

Lord of Troubled Hearts,
I can never thank you enough for those courageous words,
"Sara, God who was God two weeks ago when our son was
alive is still God today!" Those parents have planted seeds of
faith, hope, and love in the hearts of countless people across
our country. Let them return with songs of joy as you shepherd them through the valley of tears. Hug their precious
hearts close to your heart, Jesus. Bless you for sending your
angels for that old pastor who had served you so well and
wanted nothing but to see your face. Comfort this family in
a way I could not. Take their troubled hearts to your heart,
Lord of all Comfort.

Walking with Grieving Families

Grief is a universal experience. It pulls us in so many different directions as we experience conflicting emotions: faith and doubt; calm and shock; trust and anxiety; confidence and despair; peace and anger. Whereas mourning is an external process, grief is the internal process. All the emotions which are common to grief—sadness, anger, depression, loneliness— lie inside us and we may need help to express them.

Our microwave, fast-track society allows little time for grief as it shouts, "Get it over with and get on with life!" And we suppress grief and poke it down inside us as we put on a mask to show the world how strong and adjusted we are— "Laughing on the Outside, Crying on the Inside," as the popular tune of yesteryear goes. One young mother returned to work just two weeks after her young daughter was killed in a tragic accident. On her first day back, she found herself lashing out at a trusted coworker. Tears spilling from her eyes, the young mother told her friend, "That was my grief speaking."

Grief is not an illness, weakness, self-indulgence, or bad habit. It is an essential spiritual and psychological process. If we hold it in too long, we'll drown on the inside. "Grief work" is aptly named because it is work and it must be done. In a recent workshop for caregivers, Dr. Harold Ivan Smith identified the many faces of grief: exaggerated grief; inhibited grief; delayed grief; unrecognized grief; abbreviated grief; stacked grief; anticipatory grief; destructive grief; redemptive grief. I have seen all these faces of grief in my patients and their families at Tampa General Hospital, and I've also seen the physical and spiritual damage of denying these griefs. Unresolved grief can make us ill, brittle, unrelenting, depressed, and hostile to God's love and grace.

A decade ago a sixteen-year-old male entered our Emotionally Handicapped Unit. He was the son of an Air Force Colonel stationed at a nearby military base. When he was thirteen, his mother died of cancer after a prolonged time of suffering. When she died at midnight, the father left the military hospital to return home and wake up his son. "Your mother has died. Get dressed and come to the hospital with me." At the hospital the father told his son, "You have thirty minutes to say your good-byes and do your crying. After that, I never want to see you cry again over your mother!" Is it any wonder he came to our unit after suffering so many faces of grief? Grief with no closure has been called "the enemy of the living."

One does not "get over" a great grief. One can, however, with God's grace, reconcile with it. In his book, *Grief Counseling and Grief Therapy: A Handbook for the Mental Health Practitioner*, J. William Worden poses four questions that chart a person's progress:

Have you accepted the reality of the loss?

Have you experienced the pain and the grief of the loss?

Are you adjusting to the environment without the lost person or object?

Are you reinvesting your emotional energy in life?

As caregivers assisting patients and families in progressing through these stages, we need to be aware of some "Do Nots."

Do not minimize or depreciate their grief by telling them how much worse others are.

Do not spout off Scripture or pious platitudes, which grieving families are unable to bear.

Do not say, "I understand what you're going through." You don't!

Do not paint a rosy, unrealistic picture of an "all is right" future.

Do not urge them to get back into a stream of activities so they can "forget."

Do not tell a family, "This is God's will."

There are many gifts we can offer patients and families as we enter their pain without "Pollyannalizing." The greatest gift is simply the gift of yourself—availability. Let your listening heart be present with them and to them—"with-it-ness." Offer concrete help. Avoid the phrase, "If you need anything, just call." People seldom do. If you see a need, such as child care while family members are visiting their loved ones, arrange it. Shoe-leather your concerns! Often patients are medically untouchable and families, deprived of touching their loved ones, need the support of a handshake, a hug, assurance of arms tightly wound about them, or a kiss on the cheek. When you know your families, you'll know how to touch them.

Encourage spouses not to make too hasty decisions about moving or disposing of their loved one's belongings. Major decisions should be delayed if possible. Encourage family members to express their emotions honestly and freely instead of trying to be nice or acceptable. Their secrets, if they have them, are safe with you. Listen to them without hurrying them. Advise them to recall memories and live with them, not run from them. Urge them to stay with those memories until they can thank God for that person with whom they walked for a season. Reach into your experience bank for examples if they request help, but do it gently with healing intent. When you do these things, you have earned the right to point the patient or family member to the Savior who gifts us with strength and endurance.

Late in his life, Robert Frost was asked to distill the wisdom of all his years. Promptly he replied that he could do that in three words: "Life goes on!" And so it does. Family members can go on, enriched by grief's slow wisdom and the assurance that the Burden Bearer takes all our sins and grief.

Nine years ago I wrote the following words in the final chapter of my book, *Dear God, I'm Divorced!*

The pain of any loss lessens and at times disappears entirely. Yet it resurfaces briefly in unexpected moments as vividly as ever. This is not to say my grief process was unsuccessful. Rather, it says that joy and sorrow cohabit. I will never fully recover until I cross over to the Big House. There are some things our fix-it society simply can't repair. The pain, however, is now a gentle, kind pinch never quite allowing me to forget the fragility of my humanity, the vulnerability of my heart. To make peace with pain is not to deny or ease what once was. Every time I look at the tall frame of the son who most resembles his father, I am reminded briefly of what once was. But it is a joyous, peaceful remembering, though tinged with a trace of sadness. I am more gentle and patient with myself than I once was. Losses interrupt plans; they change us and alter forever the course of our lives. Grief scholar Rabbi Lindemann reminds us that it is up to us "to find a way to replace that which at first seems irreplaceable." Suffering has the possibility of teaching, tempering, and gentling as no other experience can. When we give God permission to walk by our side through this suffering, pain can be transformed into a source of new life, new direction. From the abyss, Nietzsche proclaimed, "That which does not kill you strengthens you." Hemingway declared, "Life breaks us all, but some are stronger at the broken places."

In the beautiful biblical drama of the raising of Lazarus from the dead, Jesus commanded the mourners to roll away the stone and, moments later, to unloose Lazarus's grave clothes and let him go. Not until I became a chaplain did I understand the significance of this command. How wise is our Lord in involving community to roll the stone away and release the prisoner. We are God's community. And God is still in the business of calling community to roll away the stones of grief, fear, loneliness, isolation, abandonment, and suffering through the gift of our unhurried presence. "The Lord God has given me the tongue of a teacher, that I may know how to sustain the weary with a word. Morning by morning he wakens—wakens my ear to listen as those who are taught" (Isaiah 50:4).

The apostle Paul tells us not to "grieve as others do who have no hope" (1 Thessalonians 4:13). How we bear our grief and how we minister to others in their grief is our testimony of faith.

Prayer

> "You will grieve, but your grief will turn to joy"
> (John 16:20b, NIV)

Dear Grief Bearer,
Thank you, Lord, for walking beside us in our grief, never chiding us but helping us to be strong in the broken places through the gift of your promises that joy will return. I trust you, Rock of my salvation. Help me to roll away stones of loneliness and isolation with my presence.

Assisting Families
in Saying their Good-byes

The original meaning of "good-bye" was "God be with you," or "Go with God." It was calling down a blessing on a traveler, telling him he was not alone. "Do not be afraid, for a loving Presence will accompany you on your journey." Scripture abounds with blessings, for example, this famous priestly blessing given by God to Moses, Aaron, and his sons:

> The Lord bless you and keep you; the Lord make his face to shine upon you, and be gracious unto you; the Lord lift up his countenance upon you, and give you peace. (Numbers 6:24-25)

Or this:

> The Lord himself will go before you and be with you; he will never leave you nor forsake you. Do not be afraid. Do not be discouraged. (Deuteronomy 31:8, NIV)

Our present saying, "God bless!" is another form of good-bye. We all need to learn to say our good-byes, and these begin early in life. The first day in school is a good-bye—a leaving and letting go of familiarity and security. And this process continues throughout our lives, with or without our permission. Is there any good-bye, however, that goes so deeply as death?

How do you say "good-bye" to one you love dearly? I have experienced earthly good-byes to half of my birth family: my daddy, my mama, and my younger brother. Daddy took the initiative in our earthly farewell. On my last visit with him, just before I departed, Daddy began with, "Daughter...." From early childhood he called me daughter when he wanted to impress on me some truth. He ended it with his unsurpassed wit. "I really feel sorry for those who die in the year after I do. I plan to corner that old warrior Paul and ask him about all those things I see darkly, and I expect this will take at least a year of dialogue!" Lifting himself up in his wheelchair, he then wrapped his frail arms about me and touched my cheek with his. I was but twenty-seven years old, but I can still see his sparkling eyes.

I took the initiative in saying good-bye to Mama, for she was much more reserved than Daddy and I knew it was up to me. Slipping in from Florida for an Easter visit, I knew it would be our last and so did she. A quietness of eternity had settled in her whole being. Words were few. Pulling up Daddy's old rocker, I sat by her bed all day. How I longed to tell her everything I had cradled in my heart so long, but I couldn't. Brushing back the tiny wisps of new hair that peeked from under her wig, I took my courage in hand and whispered, "Mama, soon you will be making the Great Journey." She smiled and nodded her head. "Mama, I've had lots of people mothering me all these years. I guess it took all of them! But I want you to know you are the best. I don't know how I'm going to give you up. But I do so gladly, because you are going to see Jesus and Daddy!" The radiant smile that crossed her face as she took my hand and brushed it across my cheek is etched forever in memory's tapestry.

I said good-bye to my younger brother six years later after he had battled cancer for months and months. On his last night on earth, his wife Lila was sitting with him in his hospital room. Suddenly he said, "Lila, come and sit with me on the bed." When she did, he took her hand and brushed it across her cheek, just as Mama had brushed my cheek and his cheek. He was saying, "Lila, God be with you. Let go of me and go with God." He died during the night.

Jesus so often reached out and touched those he healed. The electricity of his vibrant touch entered those who needed healing. In her book, *Praying Our Goodbyes*, Joyce Rupp gives us good advice. "We can't pry the ache out of one another but we can bless it with the touch of our hands and give it permission to go on its way."

Caregivers who have experienced significant good-byes in their own lives have a head start in ministering to families who are just beginning to say theirs. We walk the family's Emmaus road with them, listening intently for clues. We observe their family dynamics, noting the bold ones and the more reserved ones. We may feel led to nudge them, as I did a son who was busy holding his family together, and had not taken time to get closure by saying good-bye to his Dad. Some will ask us how to do it, and we can draw out experiences from our memory banks that might help them. I have sat with patients or family members and read some of the significant blessings from the Old Testament and had them repeat the blessing with me. Some have surprised and delighted me by memorizing them and using them.

This morning's mail brought a letter from my dear friend, Dr. Harold Ivan Smith, who had just buried his mother. He told of conducting her memorial service:

> I did some unusual things. Had a crown on her casket. The Nazarenes always sang, "When the battle's over, we shall wear a crown..." and then at the funeral I said, "Momma, you always talked about someday wearing a crown...and today you are." Then I took the crown from the casket spray and placed it in her hands. What a gifted good-bye for Momma! Complete with a crown. I know she loved it.

Prayer

"Blessed are those who are invited to the marriage
supper of the Lamb!"
(Revelation 19:9)

Dear Majesty in Heaven,
I have so many waiting for me in the Big House, Lord! The urge to see your face and theirs and never say good-bye again is so strong at times. But I still have work to do for you down here, walking with families and reminding them that you will go before them and be with them in all their good-byes. And that we all have a gracious invitation to the wedding supper of the Lamb! I will bless you forever.

Giving Family Members Permission to Cry

How well I remember the morning I gave a young teen permission to cry! His father was a Cherokee Indian of such stature and girth he hardly fit the small bed in Cardiac Intensive Care. He had been the driving force of his family until he was felled by a heart attack. Now he lay so silently, so still, with tubes encircling him. His wife and her two sisters stood on the right side of his bed in deep, whispered conversation. On the left side of his bed stood his fifteen-year-old son, so alone, so fragile in appearance when measured by his father's physical frame. He kept his eyes on his father's face as if to shut out all else. Suddenly his lower lip quivered and he turned from his father's bed. Quietly I moved to his side and placed a gentle hand on his shoulder, directing him out the door. His muscles quivered as he tried to hold himself together.

In a soft voice I asked him, "Has anyone given you permission to cry over your father?"

Shaking his head, he let go of that huge lump of unshed tears that had lingered so long inside his tear ducts. Sensing he needed someone to hold him, I placed my arms around him. When his body stilled, I gathered both of his hands into mine and looked him squarely in the eye.

"Son, real men do cry. Don't ever be ashamed of your tears. Please give yourself permission to cry."

After a moment or so he gave me a shy hug, straightened his shoulders, and walked back into his father's room a half head taller.

After twenty-five years spent in the company of special

needs children and adults, I have come to know the value of tears. They are not a sign of weakness, but of strength. What insane cultural messages our men have internalized! "Tears are sissy, sadness weakens. Big boys don't cry. Take it like a man!" Such myths have made emotional "Lone Rangers" of far too many men and boys as they isolate their emotions even from their family and friends, and grieve alone.

Jesus shed tears. In his gospel, John revealed a volume on the Son of Man with two words, "Jesus wept." Ever knowing he would restore his friend Lazarus to life, the Savior entered the pain and heartbreak of the two sisters when he wept with them for their brother. On another occasion, Jesus sat on a hill overlooking Jerusalem and cried out in anguish, "Jerusalem, Jerusalem…how often have I desired to gather your children together as a hen gathers her brood under her wings, and you were not willing!" (Matthew 23:37). His heart broke over this city and he wept. And he gives us permission to weep also.

Tears are like rain which cleanses and softens the earth and makes it grow green. Tears can signal the greening of our souls. They cleanse and remove toxins and hard clods of pent-up feelings from our emotional banks. They make our spirits grow upward. And if we leave them inside too long, they will drown us emotionally when we least expect it.

Inaudibly we can invite family members to cry and release the emotional dam within our encircled arms. Three years after I had experienced the dissolution of a twenty-eight-year marriage, I returned to the city where we had lived for three years. As I entered the front door of my hosts, Dale and Edie Hatch just gathered me in their arms and all three of us wept openly. "We loved you both," they sobbed. "We loved you both! Forgive us for not writing; we didn't know what to say, what to write…." Their tears shed for me and their arms about me spoke more eloquently than any word.

Just the four words, "It's okay to cry," can release a dam of unshed tears for family members suffering the wounds of loss. "I'm here with you," also conveys permission to let go of stored tears. Just being there for people, however, is your greatest gift. In one of our Clinical Pastoral Education sessions on grief, my supervisor, a former military chaplain, related a deeply moving experience.

Leaving late for a preaching engagement, I headed out on a rain-slicked road with my wife, son, and daughter. We were going on a family outing later. Visibility was limited and I misjudged the distance of an oncoming car while passing the car in front of me. Suddenly I found myself being treated for wounds in a military hospital while learning my wife was in critical condition and my children were in pediatrics, their condition not yet determined. I found a bench and sat there all alone with head in hands, trying to absorb the shock and horror.

After a few minutes, a young military chaplain came and sat on the bench with me. For the longest time he just sat there. After what seemed an eternity, he put his arm about my shoulder and muttered, "Life's a bummer!"

Chaplain Al broke down at that point in his story and wept openly before us. Then he told us he would be forever grateful to that young chaplain. "He didn't mention God. He didn't offer any pious platitudes or any explanations as to why this had happened. He just blurted out his heartcry, which was also mine in all my undoneness." That young chaplain exercised the gift of silence and "just being there."

Prayer
> *"You took our infirmities and carried our sorrows..."*
> *(Isaiah 53:4, NIV)*

O Grief Bearer,
Thank you for our tear ducts. Thank you for showing us
your tears. Savior, your heart is pierced when our heart is
pierced and you are right there with us in all our grief. Wrap
your strong arms about this frail lad who is so alone. Hold
him close so he can hear your heartbeat, and whisper in his
mother's ears how desperately he needs a hug from her.
You've promised your blessing and comfort to all who
mourn. What a promise I claim for all my patients!

Becoming Kingdom Scarecrows

Tampa General rocked with merriment on Halloween when the annual children's parade wound its way through the first floor offices and other lucrative locations. The children made out like bandits, filling their orange pails with every known goodie. There would be a surge of sugar levels in the hospital tonight! Children wore costumes of every description—pumpkins, ghosts, witches, fairies, demons, devils, kings, queens, dwarfs, animals, vegetables, and a myriad of their favorite book characters.

Creativity ran amok on this special day. Some of the children navigated IV poles that sported brightly colored streamers and humorous signs. Parents pulled their little ones on small pallets in ribbon-decked red wagons while joyous nurses carried the babies. Many of the children forgot that they had cancer and other diseases as they donned hats, caps, and wigs blossoming with buttons, bows, badges, yarn, and small signs. I was decked out as a scarecrow, with blades of straw departing at too regular intervals from my battered, broadrimmed hat.

Prancing about in the line of children, I looked at a hall clock and discovered it was 2:56. Woe be to this scarecrow! I had promised the wife of one of my patients that I would be in his room by 3:00 that afternoon. At his request, she was taking her husband home to die. Breaking from the line, I frantically dashed for the nearest elevator, completely oblivious of my ridiculous get-up. As luck would have it, of course, two doctors I knew were also going up on that elevator. Staring at me while trying to hold back their laughter, they greeted me with, "Chaplain, you have a very versatile role!"

As I huffed into the hospital room right on the dot, the wife was standing by a large suitcase. We enfolded each other in a silent bear hug, then moved toward her husband's bed, where I offered a farewell blessing. Heading for the door as tears washed down my cheeks, I was halted by her voice.

"Sara, that's the first time I've ever had a scarecrow pray for me."

If God can use a talking donkey to warn one of his disobedient servants and turn him from the path of destruction, God can surely use a scarecrow in Tampa General! Too often we are overly concerned about appearances or actions that would brand us as odd to other people. We don't want our families coming to "take us away" as did the mother and brothers of Jesus. Yet the apostle Paul, on more than one occasion declared, "We are fools for the sake of Christ..." (1 Corinthians 4:10). When we caregivers have our eyes focused on the Living Lord, and our ears attuned to his purpose for a specific patient, a purpose he expects us to fulfill, it is an honor to "suffer fools gladly for his sake."

Prayer

"Do not be afraid, little flock, for it is your Father's good pleasure to give you the kingdom."
(Luke 12:32)

Father to Little Children and Dying Patients,
Did you ever see such bravery as those moppets of all ages?
Did it remind you of the days your Beloved Son walked this planet? Thank you for jolting my memory and having that elevator right on the ground floor. That was almost a small miracle! And the funny look on those doctors' faces canceled my disappointment in leaving the parade. But most of all, I'm grateful for those words, "Sara, that's the first time I ever

had a scarecrow pray for me." I'll remember those endearing words forever! You gave me a special gift.

Now, Father, give the kingdom to these little ones today with great pleasure. Take the pain of this special one who is taking her husband home to die, and hold both of them close to your heart. Receive this husband into your kingdom, and whisper to his wife, "Fear not! I am right here beside you, pouring my love into your wounded heart." Blessed be your name!

Listening with Our Hearts

In the late 1980s an intriguing ad appeared in the Los Angeles *Times*. In a tiny block were these words, "I will listen to you 30 minutes for $5," followed by a phone number. A cub reporter, sensing a human interest item, jumped on the story and reported the ad sender received more than 100 calls the first day it appeared. The man who placed it had no degree in psychology or counseling, nor had he been to college. He just realized the desperate hunger to be listened to, and he offered a "talk cure."

"Of all the services Christians give to one another, listening is the greatest." Dietrich Bonhoeffer's words from a German prison jarred me out my tranquility. What ever happened to listening? It is the lost "L" in learning. You don't learn anything when you are talking. A Native American proverb states, "Listen or thy mouth will make thee deaf."

A chaplain friend of mine penned a book, *Who Stole the Front Porch?* Front porches with banisters and high-back rocking chairs invited conversation, socializing, high commerce, theology, sports updates, and an occasional proposal of marriage. These activities were often accompanied by a tall glass of lemonade or a long drink of cold water. Such old-fashioned togetherness has been eclipsed by hurryitis and fast-track living.

One of the popular stories of hospital life tells of two doctors meeting in the hospital corridor. The orthopedic surgeon is sympathizing with the psychiatrist, "I don't know how you can spend all your day listening to people."

The psychiatrist replies, "Who listens?"

Who, indeed? Yet what hospital patients really want is to be listened to, respected, and understood. Isn't this the cry of all humans? Why then do we not listen? Listening is hard work that calls for the expenditure of effort in concentration, the giving of undivided attention, and our ego taking a back seat. Listening takes time. It involves pauses, periods of silence while the speaker ponders and tries to put things together that they want to express. We fear silence, and want to rush in and cover it up, instead of relaxing and waiting. All too often we are just biding our time until we can take center stage. With great amusement I remember a social gathering of several faculty members at Western Carolina University. The hostess was going full speed, giving every detail of her heart surgery. My department chairperson nudged me and grumbled, "I wish she'd hurry and shut up so I can tell about my heart attack!"

Listening isn't carried on with ears alone. It involves eyes, hands, arms, feet, head, and heart. Every power of the body and mind is focused on the listening task. Every aspect of the listener communicates the message, "Tell me more. You're in the center stage of my thinking."

Some people are always talking because they never want to listen, especially to themselves. It threatens their status quo, defined as "the mess we's in." Jesus had strong words of condemnation for the Pharisees, who had well-functioning ears but refused to listen. Faulty listening habits also include trying to outguess or help the speaker with the conclusion by verbalizing what we think it is. There is the cross-examiner, who keeps interrupting and demanding details which are nonessential, thereby making the patient feel he is on trial or taking oral exams. Caregivers need to look at all of these poor listener traits and ask themselves, "How many of these hit me in the solar plexus?"

Jesus is our role model in listening with the heart. Study carefully the Emmaus road experience in Luke 24. Two disciples were heartbroken over the death of Jesus. The sun had gone out of their lives, and they were discussing the tragedy as they walked the road to Emmaus. As they were talking, Jesus himself came up and walked along with them. Caregiving is accompanying others on the footpath.

After walking with them, Jesus asked, "What are you discussing together as you walk along?" He was determined to get them talking about this event. Cleopas asked Jesus, "Are you a visitor in Jerusalem and do not know the things that have happened?" Jesus answered, "What things?" He knew they had already talked themselves out, and he could have just taken up where they left off and saved himself some time. But he knew they needed to talk. In essence he was saying what all good counselors say: "Even though I know when and why you are hurting, tell me about it."

Jesus listened intently without interruption, then taught them what the Scripture said about himself. By this time, dusk was falling, and they urged him to tarry with them. They wanted to hear more! Sitting at the table with them, he took the bread, gave thanks, broke it, and gave it to them. Where had they seen that before? Just as they recognized him, he disappeared.

"Were not our hearts burning within us while he talked with us on the road and opened the Scriptures to us?" That is our calling: to make patients' hearts burn inwardly for such fellowship with the Savior. We do that by listening as Jesus listened: with every power of our being focused on the person and his or her needs. We do that by listening without passing judgment. We do that by creating a safe, quiet, sacred space for the soul of a troubled one to come for a visit.

Caregiver, aspire to practice redemptive listening, that willingness to lose yourself in order to hear the desperate heartcry of another.

Prayer

"Listen to his voice and hold fast to him.
For the Lord is your life."
(Deuteronomy 30:20, NIV)

Listener of My Heart,

As I write this, I stand guilty before you, Lord, for speaking when I should have been listening to my patient in his distress. It takes discipline to forget my agenda or what I think my patient needs, and listen to their needs even as you listened on the Emmaus road. All of us have Emmaus roads and desperately need someone to listen as we walk those roads. You promised to set a guard on my mouth and keep watch over the door of my lips. You probably need to stuff a clean sock down my throat, too. Walk beside me and help me to be quick to listen and slow to speak. Lord, I believe!

Understanding Our Patients

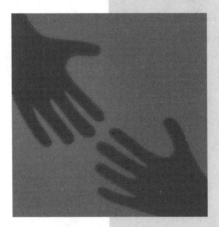

*What they're telling us in their words
and by their actions*

Addressing the Concerns of Children Facing Death

Jason, only four years young, was dying of leukemia. Nurse Gail, working the midnight shift at the hospital, tiptoed into his room and quietly did her check. Suddenly Jason threw off his sheet and blanket and popped up in the bed.

"Miz Gail, did you know I'm gonna die in a few weeks?" Dying children seem to intuitively know these things. They possess a wisdom far beyond their years.

Startled that he knew, Gail sat on the side of the bed and cradled his small hand in hers. "Jason, are you afraid to die?"

A long, grown-up minute huddled between them as Jason considered this serious question.

"No, not really, Miz Gail. You see, I'm going to see God and then turn into an angel and watch over my mommy and daddy and two-year-old sister. Right now I'm being brave for my mommy and daddy 'cause they're so scared I'm gonna die."

Having disposed of the big stuff in his life, Jason flung both arms in the air joyfully and executed a perfect somersault, landing himself right on top of Gail.

"Miz Gail, do you think we'll have to pee in heaven?"

Oh, the absolute candor of children! They wear no masks and tell it like it is—to them. In my pediatric rotation, I found children far more open and willing to talk about death than their parents were. Often the children had to turn to each other for discussion and support because parents were unwilling or forbade talk about death. Why do we exclude children from these discussions? We send them to relatives, or tell them unbelievable lies about someone going on a trip or going to sleep.

Children have large antennae that pick up far more than we suspect. They note what is being said, what is not being said, facial expressions, body language, and tone of voice. They know something is wrong, something is not being told them, and their distrust of adults multiplies when more adults tell the same cockeyed version of the story to avoid questions or further exploration. Is it any wonder that small children are afraid to go to sleep as they might not wake up? Any wonder that they express deep anxiety when a family member goes off on a trip? Their loved ones might not come back! Children then grow up with no closure on unresolved grief or nameless fears. They also wonder if they can ever trust an adult to be straightforward and honest.

Children know when the hourglass is running out. An eight-year-old asked the chaplain to help her make a list of the belongings she wanted to give to her friends because she couldn't spell the names of some of her things. "I'm dying," she said, "but my mommy won't help me. Please help me so I can get this done."

Caregivers can be listening companions for children by treating their concerns very seriously and helping them with any of their requests. This may very well include their desire for you to speak to their parents and persuade them to take their child seriously and help him or her get ready to die. I am absolutely amazed at the strength children show in handling this.

Children also need extra hugs or touch therapy from you. Unconsciously, some parents who are told of their child's critical condition may begin the process of detachment from the child because of the unbearable pain of separation. The child senses this detachment immediately but is bewildered as to its cause.

One ten-year-old who sensed his death and his parents'

inability to admit such a thing actually made an appointment with his doctor, who had an office in the hospital. The young boy came alone to the doctor's office, sat straight in the big chair across from the doctor, and announced solemnly, "I have come to talk to you about death."

A Nobel Prize in Parenthood should be awarded to a young family living in Florida's panhandle for their courage and wisdom in the death of their four-year-old Down's Syndrome daughter. The bubbly little girl knew everybody in the small community. At her death the parents asked the parish priest to invite all the children to come to the memorial service and sit in a group at the front where they could see and hear everything.

The little girl's favorite songs were played and people told warm stories about their little friend. As the children exited the front door, the priest gave each of them a brightly colored balloon to mark this celebration of their friend. On the way home from the service, the six-year-old in the family asked, "Do you think Sissy is in heaven now?" When assured that she was, he answered, "Good! I want her to be there before I let go of my balloon and send it up to her."

Immediately upon arriving home, the mother brought the two remaining children to the kitchen table. She showed them two hearts she'd made; one was huge and the other one small. Handing them the large heart, she explained, "This is your heart. It's a big, strong heart." Then she handed them the small heart, and continued, "This is your sister's heart. You see, she was born with a small heart. It was not a big strong one like yours, and it gave out on her. It was so weak it just quit beating. So you don't have to worry about your heart. It is big and strong and won't quit on you!" Lesson over, she gave them a big hug and sent them out to play. What beautiful preventive therapy, found not in a medical textbook but in a mother's heart!

Recently my beloved mentor and prayer partner, Gladys Stone, celebrated her nineteeth birthday. Festivities began early and on the night before her birthday, her grandson snuggled up to her on the host's couch. "Amah," he asked, "do you think you'll live through the night?" Somewhat startled at the question, she told him that she had every intention of doing so, with so many parties the next day. A few minutes later Brandon told her, "Amah, the reason I asked you that question was because my other three grandparents died at eighty-nine, and I wanted to be sure you're gonna make it to ninety!" Brandon had graduated from a university, so children of all ages have honest concerns about death, and they deserve straightforward and honest answers from us.

Parents need not go into lengthy explanations, but they do need to answer each question simply and honestly, using age-appropriate language. Impress upon your parents, "If you want your child's trust, never tell him or her anything you will have to retract or take back later." Encourage parents and family members to utilize their church or public library for excellent books on explaining death to a child.

A young mother in one of my conferences told me of taking her young son to his great-grandmother's funeral. "She was ninety-five and the matriarch of our family. Our son had spent many fun-filled days and nights with her. He also noticed her gradual decline and understood that her body had just worn out, so we felt right in allowing him to go with us for the final good-bye to Mam Maw."

When he saw his Mam Maw in the casket, he looked a bit puzzled by the satin and lace quilting that covered most of her body. After a second look, he announced solemnly, "At least God let Mam Maw keep her head!"

Prayer

> *"From the lips of children and infants*
> *you have ordained praise."*
> *(Psalm 8:2, NIV)*

Shepherd of Little Children,
O, the faith of these small wonderments of your creation!
You have told us their angels go in and out of your Presence.
How we need their honesty and forthrightness. Jason's small
words, "Right now I'm trying to be brave for my mommy
and daddy," tore a big hole in my heart. Cradle his small
body in your strong arms, Good Shepherd. And Jesus, I'm
with Jason. Being still a child at heart, I hope we don't have
to pee in heaven!

Why?

Why? Why? Why? This seemingly unanswerable question has been the heartcry of generation upon generation. In the Old Testament, psalmists, prophets, and kings grappled with it. It is not easy to surrender to God that which we do not understand. Job asked again and again the "why" of suffering, especially for good people who love God and do good. Multitudes of saints have spent hours upon their knees seeking an answer to this question. Even our Savior, in his most alone hour on earth, cried out, "My God, my God, why have you forsaken me?" Every professional or volunteer caregiver will be asked this question by heartbroken families. How it steadies and sustains me to know that disappointment in God need not be a terminal condition!

I can still hear the piercing cry of one whose husband had taken his life. They were childhood sweethearts from Michigan who had been married for sixty years. Upon retirement they moved to the sunny shores of Tampa to escape bitter winters. He made the coffee and toast for her each morning, reminding her of all the years she'd risen before dawn to make breakfast and see him off to work.

Their golden years were interrupted when a deadly cancer struck him. He had been in the hospital for a long time, then finally returned home. Their son had come from California for a much awaited visit. As usual, Dad made the coffee and toast the next morning as soon as he heard his son stirring. When the son entered the kitchen, a loud gun blast shattered his family's life forever. Rushing to the garage workshop, he found his dad lying in a pool of blood, with half of his face gone. His mother was in the kitchen by now, and he hurried in to prevent her from entering the garage.

I met the family in the Quiet Room at the hospital. The husband was comatose, barely alive in the Emergency Room. Two of the wife's sisters were huddled together on a couch, and the wife was seated on another couch across the room. Her son was seated in a chair beside her. I always try to observe the facial expressions and seating arrangements of family members, as they give me powerful clues. A caring nurse came into the room and told them they could see their family member if they desired.

The sisters announced that they would go, but under no circumstance was the wife to go in. The son followed them out, stating that he was going to the cafeteria. I moved to the wife's side and held her hand lightly, realizing she was still in shock. We sat quietly for a few minutes, then suddenly she turned to me and said, "I want to go and see my husband. I need to, but I'm afraid. And I don't want to go with my sisters. What should I do?"

When I realized that the question was not rhetorical, I answered, "I cannot presume to tell you what to do. Only you can decide that. I do know family members who chose not to go, and then they regretted it because they didn't speak their farewells in private. They had difficulty getting closure later on."

After a moment's hesitation, she looked at me and asked, "Chaplain, would you go with me?"

"Certainly," I said. "And I'll ask Big John, my favorite orderly, to go with us. We will be on each side of you, holding you tightly until you return."

With firm resolve, she arose. I collected Big John en route, and he held her arm gently. Upon entering the curtained cubicle she almost sank to her knees, but we held her firmly. After a minute she indicated that she wanted to go to her husband's side, so we helped her over there. Her eyes focused on his face swathed in white as she spoke to him.

"Why did you do it? Why did you leave me? Why? Why? We had so much to live for! I would have taken care of you for as long as God gave us together, just as you have taken care of me. Didn't you know that?" As she raged, wept, and became tender with her husband, we removed our support and stood just behind her. Finally spent, she whispered, "I'm ready to go now." Her husband died later that night.

The whys of pain and suffering have been shrouded in mystery since time began. If God chooses not to audibly answer this mystery, we caregivers would be presumptuous to try and answer this agonizing, searing question in the hearts of others. I've seen irreparable harm done by caregivers spouting out glib answers.

Many whys have come into my own life. Later, as I reflected on them, I realized that they were more of a how than a why. "How will I ever get through this experience, Lord? I am your child, so tell me how! I read your promise in your Word:

When you pass through the waters, I will be with you;
and through the rivers, they shall not overwhelm you;
when you walk through fire you shall not be burned,
and the flame shall not consume you.
For I am the Lord your God,
the Holy One of Israel, your Savior! (Isaiah 43:2,3)

I believe that promise. Would you show me how to pass through those rivers and flames as you hold my hand? I won't make it on my own!"

As a result of these experiences, I remain silent on the whys and focus on how to help my patients and their families get through this valley of the shadow of death without stalling out. In his book, *How Can It Be All Right When Everything Is All Wrong?* Lewis Smedes says, "When you hurt with hurting people, you are dancing to the rhythms of God." How so? With your quiet presence, a gentle touch of your hand, and the offer of a listening heart as patients or family members run the gamut of bewilderment, confusion, disbelief, fear, anger, helplessness, self-pity and self-blame. Do not be put off by their raging or storming at you. Stay with them, remembering you are not the target! And God, the Supreme Sufferer who is also the Supreme Comforter, will use you to comfort those who have been torn apart by life's hurts.

As an act of worship, we can bring all of our whys and hows to the One who also asked why.

Prayer

"Even though I walk through the valley of the shadow of death, I will fear no evil, for you are with me."
(Psalm 23:4, NIV)

Lord over Death,
Job asked, "Who then can understand...?" We cannot understand these things, Jesus. We can only hold on to the hem of your garment and cry out, "Have mercy on me." I place this dear wife and mother with all her whys in your strong arms. She is one of your precious lambs; hold her tightly. Comfort her with your own tears.

Allowing Patients to "Own" their Feelings

Three months after her husband's funeral, a young widow blurted out, "I'm so mad at my husband for up and dying and leaving me to raise three young children, I could go out to the cemetery, dig him up, and wring his neck!" Horrified at her words and her seeming betrayal of her husband's love, she asked herself, "Where did these words come from?" Where, indeed? These brutally honest words signaled the anguish and abandonment she felt in her heart.

How often our feelings and emotions catch us by surprise! A few snatches of a certain melody can produce somersaults of joy or a basin of tears. We can laugh and cry at the same time. Feelings can be our friend and our foe. They cannot be deposited into the out basket of our lives without serious consequences. When we fear our feelings we actually fear ourselves, for feelings provide us with information about ourselves, even though we may not want to deal with that information. Feelings are legitimate and are to be confronted, honored, and respected. Even if they are negative, they are not to be suppressed and run underground. John Calvin once described feelings as, "an anatomy of all parts of the soul."

You and I can actually thank God for our feelings. Whether they make us comfortable or uncomfortable, they remind us that we are still involved in living. They also signal us that grief work isn't yet done. Expressing our feelings is the path to emotional and spiritual wholeness. Ignoring feelings of inner unrest, anger, turmoil, tension, and sadness can bring illness in our bodies and spirits.

Early one morning I was making my way to the cafeteria for

breakfast after sixteen hours of Emergency Room on-call when my beeper screeched. The charge nurse answered my return call. "Chaplain, come quickly! We have an overdosed patient who attempted suicide. She's yelling, cursing, tearing up the place, and disturbing everybody in ER even though we have her in restraints."

As the charge nurse walked me to the patient's cubicle in ER, she continued, "The patient lost her eleven-year-old daughter to leukemia a year and a half ago. This is the patient's third suicide attempt."

Seldom have I seen such uninhibited rage and hostility. "What the hell are you doing here? I didn't ask for any chaplain! Go away. I hate God! I hate God!" Had I tried to touch her, she would have decked me and I would have been on a gurney, too. "God allowed my daughter to die and I must go where she is to take care of her. God sure as hell isn't going to take care of her. He let her die!"

In a drugged fog, she continued to pitch about and swear against God. I agitated her further by interrupting her tirade with my words, "Life isn't fair." (Did my fellow chaplains ever make mincemeat of those words and of me at our next group meeting!)

How long does grief last? This mother had stalled out in the anger stage, but I could not allow her to disturb and upset all the other patients in ER. Drastic measures were in order. When I entered her cubicle, a nurse took off her arm restraints. Still standing near the middle of her bed, I asked her in a stern voice if she wanted the nurse to return and put on her arm restraints again. She shook her head vigorously.

"Then I suggest you calm down and allow me to help you back under the sheet." Only then did I move toward the head of the bed and put out my hand. After I'd helped her down under the sheet, I gave her a back door pat on the shoulder. Standing by her gurney for a few seconds, I smiled and rested my soul. This was not the time to say anything like, "Our Father lost a child, too." When my beeper shrieked again, the patient reached over and brushed my hand. "Thank you for coming," she said quietly.

Moving on to the next call, I asked myself, "Where is her anger coming from?" I suspected that much of her anger was directed toward her daughter for leaving her, but it is unacceptable to be angry with your daughter who is now dead. Hence, she transferred most of the anger to God. He could take it! Anger is a secondary emotion, never a primary one. It is fueled by other emotions. The two emotions that drive anger are hurt and fear. When we are deeply hurt by someone or something, we defend ourselves from further injury by displaying anger. This mother was hurt deeply when her daughter died, and targeted her anger at God for "letting" her child die. As a general rule, "Where there is hurt, there is heat." The deeper the pain, the hotter and more sustained the anger. Such was this mother's rage.

After a few crash landings, I have learned not to deny patients their anger, even if it is directed toward me. If I do so, I may be blocking the only road of communication to God that is open to them right then. Resentment, frustration, and anger may be the only springboard by which they can leap to God, as did many of the prophets and psalmists of old when their anger abated. In his provocative and indispensable little book, *May I Hate God?* Pierre Wolff states, "If we cannot tell everything to our best friend, Abba, our Father in Heaven, to whom can we tell it? Absolutely nobody." Every caregiver should have this little volume on his or her library shelf.

I have found that if I remain calm and try to understand, not judge a patient when he ventilates hostility and rage, the patient no longer feels alienated and usually reduces his anger. Nurses come by more often and he no longer feels abandoned by God and man. The patient removes his mask and faces reality with more courage and certainty.

I make a yearly pilgrimage through the psalms, reading each one in five different translations. No wonder this is the favorite book in the Bible for patients, a fundamental source of spiritual support! Every human response to life's ups and downs is recorded in these 150 psalms. They are earthy, rough, honest, true, passionate, personal responses to God, devoid of "churchy language." Patients gasp in surprise when they hear some of the strong language. "These dogs, hotheads, bunch of liars are out to swallow me. Their teeth are sharp as spears, their tongues like swords. Snatch off their beards, pull out their hair, smash their teeth! Let death seize them, cut them down in their prime, let them go to the grave alive."

Those psalmists were passionate for God in moments of praise, anger, and lament. "Where are you, God? Why have you forsaken me? I am in deep trouble. I scream out to you night and day. Are you deaf? Do you realize what's going on, Lord? I think of you, God, and moan, overwhelmed with longing for your help. I can't sleep unless you act. I am too distressed to pray."

How those psalmists of old mirror my emotions and feelings! Their passion, their anger, the potency of their words are mine, too. I weep, scream, and shout with them. The immediacy of their sorrow becomes my sorrow. When the furies have me by the hair, I shut my door, put the *1812 Overture* on my stereo, and read some of those psalms at the top of my voice. What sanity savers they are!

How can you help patients "own" their feelings without fear of censure? Encourage them to befriend their feelings rather than fight or suppress them. Read them one of those expressive psalms. Remind angry or sad patients, "You can tell God about this. You can yell and scream. God can take it and you'll feel much better." Teach them to say, "God I'm really angry with you! I'm disappointed with you and am at the end of my rope."

Directing feelings toward God, even when people are angry, helps remove scales from their eyes. Suggest they write a letter to God telling him everything in their hearts. Encourage them to be specific in identifying their grievances. Then ask them if they can remember a time in the past when God was helpful to them. Have them describe that time in great detail. With their permission, share an experience of anger with God from your own life and how you worked through it. Help them find a good listener or support group. Networking is an invaluable tool of caregivers. Know where resources are available.

Above all, provide a fertile, safe climate in which they can honestly "own" their feelings without any hint of censure or shock on your part. To do so requires that you, the caregiver, return to your own brokenness and undoneness before God and remember how God restored and renewed you. In God's timing, you will be ready to share the warmth of his love and acceptance, and your redeemed scars will bring healing to patients and families.

Prayer

> *"O Lord, do not be far away! O my help,*
> *come quickly to my aid."*
> *(Psalm 22:19)*

Compassionate Father,
Every word I cry out, you hear and you act. How precious
are your promises even when I am mad or at odds with you!
Speak love to my patients who feel abandoned by you and
by their families. Help me communicate your unconditional
acceptance of them by my word and by my touch. Spill your
amazing grace over into my heart and theirs, Abba Father.
Bend down and whisper grace to the young mother who has
given up on you.

Coping with Attention-Seeking Patients

One of the most fascinating stories of the New Testament tells of Jesus finding his way to the Pool of Bethesda, Home for the Incurables. Here the lame, blind, crippled, deaf, palsied, and all who were shells of wretchedness and despair awaited the yearly visitation of an angel who came down and stirred up the pool. He who reached the pool first was healed.

Jesus moved unhurriedly among the mats, seeking the most helpless invalid. He stopped at the mat of a man who had been at the pool for thirty-eight years. Looking into the man's eyes, Jesus asked a simple question, "Do you want to be healed?" For years this question troubled me. Why else had he been at the pool for thirty-eight years? Certainly he wanted to be healed! Or did he?

Why, he was Kingpin of the Invalids, receiving sympathy, recognition, and adulation for holding the longevity record at the pool. Were he healed, he would have to change his lifestyle. He would have to rise up and take responsibility for himself without the adulation of his cheering squad. Did he dare risk such a drastic change after making friends with his invalidism? Knowing all these things about the man, Jesus invited him with a simple command to leave behind all those securities. "Get up, take up your mat (the chief symbol of his identity) and walk."

In our Clinical Pastoral Education case history discussions, we often ask each other, "What is the payoff for this patient's illness? Why does the patient take to his bed and love it?" Coping with attention-seeking patients is one of our greatest frustrations. It often requires the wisdom of Solomon, which we don't have.

One of my female patients devoted herself to "aggravation

grief." She was aggravated at everything, especially the way Tampa General Hospital was run, and she wasted no time in fertilizing her long list and daily feeding it to the nurses, technicians, and chaplain. All I wanted to do was loudly yell, "Grow up!" at her. Instead, I told her on my third visit I could no longer come by unless she reported at least one good thing before she fired her negative missiles. Jesus reminded us more than once that what gets our attention gets us. "As people think in their hearts, so they are" (Proverbs 27:19, my paraphrase).

My first goal for her treatment plan was *refocusing*. During her two-week stay, she progressed to a daily list of five good things. Early in the morning, before she stockpiled her ammunition, I would march into her room with a big "I dare you" smile plastered on my face. Seating myself at the head of her bed, I would take her hand and say, "Tell!" When she began her gripe list, I quietly withdrew my hand, a fact that did not escape her attention. Her gripe list became shorter, and after a week I invited her to join me in prayer for her healing. She accepted.

J's best friend, who daily endured a misery visit, called me aside one day and gave me the clue for which I had been searching. "J is in middle management and is used to barking orders and seeing them carried out by disgruntled subordinates. She thrives on her need to control. Our company is now downsizing and deep down inside her, I believe J fears a pink slip because her incivility has been documented and recorded in her employment file."

This revelation brought me to my knees in the chapel and changed my attitude from endurance to acceptance and affirmation of my patient. She sensed that and began to find more positive and acceptable ways of gaining attention. Nurses inwardly cheered when the patient bade me a teary farewell after two weeks. Even they had to admit that J had begun to thank them instead of complaining all the time. J's words, "You cared for me, didn't you?" were my reward.

Caregivers, don't give up! Remember those attention-getting surface behaviors are merely symptoms of a deeper inner need, a fear, or a gaping wound that has not been addressed. Be bold but compassionate as you practice selective attention, short-circuiting the patient's griping and bullying to get at the root problem, which is usually a spiritual one. In this process, refocus your patient on positive ways to get attention. Make a list for yourself of behaviors you would like to encourage and ways you might do that. Catch the patient off guard with a question such as, "What has been the happiest day in your life?" Urge them to detail that day for you. All of this requires "on your knees" patience.

In a longer term relationship with a patient, you might use four questions to facilitate refocusing:

Do you want to be healed?

Can you identify some destructive behaviors that are delaying your healing?

What do you intend to do about these behaviors?

Would you like me to help you formulate a plan of action?

Prayer

"Whatever is true, whatever is honorable, whatever is just, whatever is pure, whatever is pleasing, whatever is commendable, if there is any excellence and if there is anything worthy of praise, think about these things."
(Philippians 4:8)

Dear Repairer of our Hearts,
I'm going to have to do some plowing up, some weeding out before I call these praiseworthy qualities mine. Forgive me,

Jesus, for just enduring this patient, for taking no joy in her that first week and for just wanting to shout, "Grow up!" You probably want to shout that to me in my stubborn stances. Thank you for looking deep in J's heart and knowing what the problem was. Lord Jesus, I know about the "failure to thrive" syndrome in neglected children, but adults can also suffer "failure to thrive." I praise you for the insights her dear friend gave me and for your strong nudges reminding me I was part of the problem. Repair her broken walls, refocus her on you, the source of nobility and rightness. I love you, Lord, for putting up with me and reshaping me with each of these hard experiences at Tampa General.

Learning
and Growing
Together

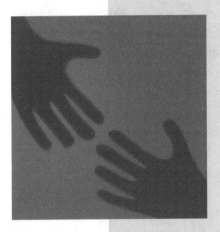

Sharing feelings, spirituality, concerns

Symbols of Faith

Elsie was a quiet oasis to whom I came for renewal and strength at the times when fatigue and anger threatened to undo me. Often she reminded me of how radically God loves each of us.

"We are wrapped in the everlasting arms of God," she told me on one memorable visit, "and each dawn is a gift as God waits to move us into a new day. Sara, would you do me a big favor when you go home tonight? I know we've already prayed, but light a candle for me tonight and say a small prayer that my faith won't sink during the long night hours. I'll rest a lot better tonight if I knew you'd done that."

Light a candle for me! In the early church Christians would stop by the church to pray and light a candle, which they took home to light their hearths and their lamps. Memories of lighting candles in churches across Europe and feeling the kinship of faith overwhelmed me as I drove homeward across Tampa Bay. How these precious symbols of faith and hope, these simple rituals, bind my patients' hearts together with God!

In pain, suffering, despair, hope, joy, and celebration, these symbols of hope glue us together. There was a grieving father who crafted a grotto in his garden while he talked and listened to God. For another family, the anointing of their son with oil and their prayer for his ultimate healing, even as they saw him enter eternity's borders, served to knit our souls together.

The Holy Scriptures, the Communion Cup and the Bread of God's Presence, a rosary, a cross, a prayer book, all bring a healing balm to both troubled and joyful hearts, and remind us that we are not alone on this planet. Let these holy things touch you and return the blessing to your patients.

When you enter a patient's room, be very observant for these tangible symbols of faith: a Bible; a cross; rosary beads; a devotional book; sacred music being played; or a religious TV program. Invite the patient to share with you the meaning of this symbol. A simple question often elicits positive responses: "What has comforted and sustained you the most during your hospital stay?" Or, "Tell me about your family's rituals of faith," will also open doors. Above all else, when you meet the "Elsies" whose radiant faith has nurtured you, tell them how much they have encouraged, enriched, and blessed you. Tell their families, too. To know they have blessed you carries them through those long nights of waiting. When invited, share your symbols of faith and your family rituals with them. I never tire of exchanging symbols of hope and blessing with my patients and their families.

A cardinal rule for all chaplains in our hospital: never diminish or take away your patients' rituals of faith. It is also a cardinal rule for all caregivers.

Prayer

"By faith…"
(Hebrews 11:8)

Precious Lord,
I'm here with lighted candle in your Presence. Bless your child, Elsie, who lives by faith. Make her night watch a joyful communion with you. And give us more Elsies at Tampa General!

Despair

There are some experiences that touch your life forever, and I had one such this morning. No one had prepared me for a "Call it!" No one told me about this trauma, and my first experience with it shook me to my toes. A Code Blue wailed early this morning while I was still chaplain-on-call, signaling a life-threatening situation. When I arrived, the team was working on a patient whose heart had arrested. I stood to the side in awe at such precision, such team concentration. Every member knew his or her assigned role.

No method was left untried for almost ten minutes. When extended use of the paddles did not alter the flat line on the monitor, the doctor in charge finally spoke the words, "Call it," while noting the time on the chart. Wordlessly the team dispersed with the agony of loss written on their faces and in their eyes. Such despair! I knew none of the team, hence I was unaware of their belief system. Where is their chaplain? I longed to move among them, touch them individually on the arm or shoulder, and whisper, "You did everything you could! You did everything you could!" Instead, I walked with the charge doctor to break the news to the waiting husband.

I felt the same deep agony the first time I entered ICU at Bangalore Baptist Hospital in India. A little boy had just died, and his Hindu mother, a second wife, was wailing loudly to her gods. "Why did you have to take my little boy? You could have taken all three daughters and left my little boy, but you took him. Why my son? Why did you snatch him from me? Why?" She then fell across his still-warm body, covered it with kisses, and fought off any nurse who tried to approach her. I stood there speechless and helpless as a native chaplain took my hand and prayed softly.

Seldom have I seen a despair deeper than that of this Indian mother! What will I do with this pervasive despair in my own heart and brain cells? "Do not, therefore, abandon that confidence of yours; it brings a great reward. For you need endurance..." (Hebrews 10:35–36). I wasn't sure I had any confidence left to throw away until I turned again to the pages of the Old Testament. Then I remembered that I was in good company.

Many prophets—Moses, Elijah, and Jeremiah, among them—had lost their confidence and begged God to kill them. Jeremiah complained to God that he was sick and tired of bearing only bad news to Judah. He seemed always to be in danger from political and religious leaders who were angry because of his messages. He even told God he would quit, resign if he could. "The word of the Lord has become for me a reproach and derision all day long. If I say 'I will not mention him, or speak any more in his name,' then within me there is something like a burning fire shut up in my bones..." (Jeremiah 20:8–9). Despite all, he concluded God was his strength, fortress, and refuge in times of distress. Humbly he asked God to correct him in gentleness, not in anger lest he be reduced to nothing.

My favorite passage on how God cures our despair is recorded in 1 Kings 19, the matchless account of God's dealings with Elijah when he was depressed, burned out, and feeling he was all alone in his love for God. God ministered first to his need for food and then for rest in the form of deep sleep. He went on to show Elijah his power over nature, then appeared to him in a gentle whisper. He allowed Elijah to vent the negative feelings that had consumed him, and next gave him specific duties which would reconfirm his calling. Only then did he remind Elijah that he was not alone, that there were 7,000 other believers in Israel who had not bowed to Baal. Lastly he gave him a helper, Elisha, to bear the burden of caring for Israel.

Despair is a signal to begin taking better care of yourself, to look inward and take inventory of your physical, mental, emotional, and spiritual levels. What are you doing to nurture yourself and to maintain balance in these areas? Check your hunger, fatigue, and sleep levels. God expects you to take care of your body, his dwelling place, his home within you. Are you treating your body shabbily? "We are God's work of art, created in Christ Jesus for good works" (Ephesians 2:10, my paraphrase).

Confront the "self" that is buried deep within protective walls and smooth defenses. To be any good to anyone, you must first listen to yourself. What is the source of this despair you are feeling? Investigate it. Are you angry, disappointed that God did not act when and how you expected? Don't run from this feeling, as Elijah did. Rather, remind yourself that God's tremendous strength is just as available today as it was to Elijah, a man subject to the same emotions and passions you have.

Embrace the pain and aloneness as you withdraw to meditate on Scripture passages which reveal God's personal touch in dealing with his distressed children. Let those passages shape your heart with compassion and understanding. Turn your distress over to God, who completely understands your despair and any circumstance which might have brought it about. Let God speak to your troubled heart and give you grace through this despair. Reaffirm God's calling in your life and the resources he has so generously provided. Like Jeremiah, humbly ask him to correct you in gentleness, "not in your anger, or you will bring me to nothing" (Jeremiah 10:24).

Finally, ask yourself, "Am I working *for* God or am I working *with* God?" It makes all the difference in the world. When you merely work for God, you experience the fatigue, despair, and resentment that employees often feel toward their employer. When you co-labor with God, watching what he is doing and joining him in his work, you mount up with enthusiasm and joy at the privilege of cooperating with him.

Prayer

"Do not hide your face from me. Do not turn your servant away in anger, you who have been my help. Do not cast me off, do not forsake me, O God of my Salvation."
(Psalm 27:9)

O Father of the Despairing,
How I wish I could have shared this prayer of assurance with the Code Blue team! Protect them, Almighty God, from anxiety, and show your love to each of them. Savior, send someone to offer your hope to the Hindu mother who refused to be consoled. Thank you for your amazing grace in our despair. When I've been with you ten thousand years, it will still amaze me, Father, that you could care so much for me.

Laughter

Faith, hope, and hilarity! Love and laughter. Caregivers with these qualities are worth far more than gold or silver, for the gift of laughter makes many unbearable things bearable. "Lighten up and let your hilarity genes run amok" is sane advice for both caregivers and patients.

Laughter is the safety belt of the nervous system. He who laughs lasts! The most wonderful sound in my ears at Tampa General is pealing laughter floating from patients' rooms. My heart is still laughing at one episode I called "The Honeymoon Elevator." A couple who had gone together all through high school but married other people had again found each other in the autumn years of their lives. They had planned a quiet wedding before he came down with a debilitating disease and entered the hospital. Despite all, the glow of the future shone brightly in their eyes, and they asked me to reserve the chapel and make arrangements for their wedding.

I was off and running, engaging the chaplains' calypso combo, decorating the chapel, and rounding up guests from favorite staff members, including my mentor, Sara. It was a three-handkerchief ceremony sprinkled with touches of laughter. Wedding news travels fast, and a small group of onlookers wished them well as the bride and groom, in his wheelchair, headed for "The Honeymoon Elevator." It proved to be an exciting trip!

Someone had spilled a puddle of water from a vase of flowers, and a very expectant mother boarded the elevator on the second floor and unknowingly stood right in the puddle of water. At the third floor a nurse's aide joined them. En route to the next floor, the aide stared down at the puddle of water and back up at the very expectant mother.

"Oh my God! Her bag of water has burst. We've got to get her to obstetrics fast!"

By the time the detour was completed, the bride and groom arrived at his room in high hilarity. As the bride's mother, two attendants and I toasted the happy pair, the groom quipped, "Were we society people, this wedding would have made exciting headlines: 'The Groom Went Back to Bed; The Bride Went Home'!"

On another hilarious occasion, laughter spilled from a ninety-year-old patient's room when he confessed he had stolen a little kiss from the night nurse. His wife, of the same age, was highly indignant about this until the day nurse chortled, "Honey, be thankful your husband can still pucker up!"

Norman Cousins first drew our attention to the healing power of laughter in his best-seller, *Anatomy of an Illness as Perceived by the Patient*. Since then, volumes have been written on patients who have laughed their way back to health. Mirth is often called "internal jogging" in which heart rate is increased, respiration is amplified, and oxygen exchange is expanded. Laughter is a "natural high therapy."

A patient with a sense of humor doesn't waste time and energy trying to be perfect, or hiding anger and frustration by sublimating it. Instead, they can deal with a greater number of problems, learning to roll with the punches and bounce back much sooner than patients who take themselves too seriously and internalize every setback as failure. When my patients can laugh at themselves, they become more candid and self-accepting, which increases their self-esteem and popularity with other patients and the staff. The same holds true for caregivers.

It is suggested that the average American laugh fifteen or more times each day. How can we encourage our patients to be more joyful and take themselves less seriously? One somewhat zany chaplain of my acquaintance carries about a brightly colored sign with the question, "Have you gotten your fifteen laughs today?" We can encourage patients to surround themselves with healthy, fun-loving friends who fill them with hope, joy, and laughter. On rare occasions I have spoken with family members about "gloom and doom" visitors or relatives who agitate and have a negative effect on the well-being of the patient.

Clergy and volunteers must have deep respect for the patient and their belief system, never insulting it with uncalled-for humor. This does not mean, however, that we must enter the patient's room with an, "I've come to help you cross the bar" countenance. At Tampa General, I do not wear a white coat as I did in India. Always I am clothed in "flowers of the field" colors. Over and over patients tell me how much it means to them for me to bring "cheer through the door" of their somewhat sterile environment. The writer of Proverbs declares, "A happy heart makes the face cheerful" (Proverbs 15:13, NIV). Happy clothes do the same.

In "A Salute to Laughter" in *Christian Ethics Today*, Dr. Foy Valentine shares some wise perceptions on humor and laughter:

> Humor, it seems to me, is God's great gift to a species prone to failure, misery, depression, wrath, remorse, sickness, disease, gout, cataracts, the common cold, war, cruelty, cancer, poverty, pain, exploitation, prejudice, hunger, pride, abuse, torture, violence, and death. If you ask me who could laugh in the face of such adversities, then I would like to ask you who could keep his head above water at all without the life raft of laughter to cling to in those wild waters?

Prayer

"A glad heart makes a cheerful countenance.
A cheerful heart has a continual feast."
(Proverbs 15:13,15)

Dear Father of Laughter,
I'm sure that all of my disasters, most of them self-inflicted,
have given you both a merry heart and a sad heart, too,
Father. Bless and keep the merry hearts of the honeymoon
couple, who are defying earthly odds in faith as they live and
enjoy one day at a time. Lift up your countenance on them,
and gift them with your peace. I love you, precious Savior.
The new wine of your presence surrounded them in the
chapel today. You save us from ourselves with your love and
laughter when we take ourselves too seriously. Thank you,
Blessed Redeemer.

Thanking God in All Circumstances

The most arresting blue eyes greeted me as I met this spirited hospice patient. A fellow chaplain had invited me to accompany him on his weekly visit to the patient's home. Suffering from Lou Gehrig's crippling disease, the patient had to be recertified three times as hospice appropriate, as he refused to die in any of those six-month time frames. He greeted us from his bed in the middle of the living room.

"Chaplain," he said, "I'm an old reprobate who's wasted too much of his life and who should have died long ago. But God has seen fit to keep me on this earth. I don't know why, because for years I drank and caroused and did my body in. Now one of the local Alcoholics Anonymous chapters meets right here in my living room every Monday night, and some of my former drinking cronies surround my bed with energy and humor as they bring the world and God to me."

His wife beamed her love to him as he spoke, and called attention to an attractive screen covered with dozens of snapshots of family and friends. Nothing would do but to capture my likeness on Polaroid and add it to the collection.

When my chaplain friend signaled a departure sign, his patient said, "One more thing, Chaplain. I want you to hear this. I thank God for everything he's given me. I thank God for everything he's taken away. I thank God for everything he's left me! Blessed be his name forever."

What an amazing statement, "I thank God for everything he's left me!" It put a halo on my day. Sometimes we thank God for what he's given us. Seldom do we thank him for what he's taken away. And rarest of all is to thank him for what he's left us. When the patient said that, he took his wife's hand and looked right into her eyes. So powerful were his emotions that I wanted to tiptoe right out the door without another word being spoken.

"Give thanks in all circumstances. In everything give thanks. Rejoice in the Lord always" (1 Thessalonians 5:18, Philippians 4:4, NIV). How often I, and a million more, have wrestled with these words from that old warrior, Paul! "Give thanks in everything" and "Rejoice always"? Surely you jest, Paul! Yet that little book of Philippians, written from a prison cell in Rome, is full of joy. The words "joy" or "rejoice" appear fourteen times in four chapters.

It finally dawned upon me that I did not have to be thankful for every circumstance or for everything that happened to me. Rather I was to give thanks in all of it. That little word *in* made a whale of a difference. Because God was right there beside me in every circumstance, I could give thanks. Again, I could not rejoice for everything that happened to me, but I could rejoice in the Lord always because he will never leave me or forsake me. Despite my mumblings and grumblings, I always return to the source of my joy, Jesus Christ!

What a joy-bringer is the patient whose bed is their tabernacle of praise! May his tribe increase!

Prayer

"At midnight I rise to give you thanks."
(Psalm 119:62, NIV)

Blessed and Only Ruler,
I praise and thank you, Lord, for this beautiful witness of your amazing grace. I shudder to think how most of us would react to being imprisoned in that bed twenty-four hours a day. How fortunate are those who come every

Monday night and surround this man's bed with joy! They are the receivers in the same way I was today. Bless this precious couple with the Spirit of counsel and power. Shepherd of my heart, I do thank you for all the things you have left me. I rejoice in your love!

A Praying Heart

Something, I know not what, compelled me to return to the Pediatrics unit, even though the dusk of a winter's day was calling me homeward across the bridge to St. Petersburg. All was still in the adolescence wing. While I was moving through the younger children's wing, I heard deep, muffled sobbing. A young father was sitting, head in hands, by a tall crib which held his son. The son lay asleep, both legs bandaged and in traction. Although fearful of disturbing his privacy, I sensed the man's great need. Moving to his side, I touched his back lightly and sat in the chair beside him in silence, as did the friends of Job. (This appeared to be the only comforting thing they did for Job.)

Soon the young father found his voice, and poured out deep anguish for his young son. Some ten minutes later he asked, "Will you pray for my son and our family?" After we had both prayed, he startled me with a new question. "Chaplain, do any of your patients pray for you?"

My words faltered as a lump rose in my throat. "I haven't been here too long, but none of my patients have prayed for me in my presence. Some tell me that they pray for me."

"Chaplain, you move about in a hostile environment of germs, death, and turmoil every day. Your patients should pray for you just as you pray for them! You need their prayers for your protection. Could we bow our heads again? This time I'm going to pray for you!"

Now I know what compelled me to return to Pediatrics.

Prayer from the heart is the greatest untapped resource in Christendom! Do we really believe, with James, that the prayer of a righteous person is powerful and effective? Many doctors today are prescribing prayer in large doses. Family physician Dr. Walt Larimore states, "Not praying for a patient who wants it is like withholding an antibiotic. Prayer costs nothing and has no side effects." He credits God as the Great Physician: "I come to work each day and he lets me see him work."

In a national survey of family physicians, ninety-nine percent believe that personal prayer, meditation, and other spiritual and religious practices can speed or help medical treatment of ill people. A 1995 study at Dartmouth Medical School found that among patients who had undergone elective heart surgery, the "very religious" recovered three times as fast as those patients who were not.

Sadly, the number of times we chaplains prayed in our group settings could be counted on one hand, with fingers left over. One of those times occurred when a fellow chaplain's wife was gravely ill. In my intern training at a large university hospital in a different state, we never prayed. The explanation given me proved unsatisfactory: "We have such a diversity of faith among chaplains that offering prayer would cause controversy."

I have problems with canned prayers or vain repetitions, but many were the times I felt such need for prayer in difficult situations and precarious decision making that I wanted to say, "Could we please pray about this?" At other times, God was so obviously present among us, I wanted to rise and ask, "Could we give God a big round of applause?" How can God's mantle of protection cover our hospitals if chaplains are too busy or too afraid of controversy to praise and petition our Lord, Creator of the universe—and of us?

I well remember collapsing in my home one night and later being taken to the hospital, where life-saving emergency surgery was performed, removing many feet of intestine. Battered, ill, and bruised, I remained a week in intensive care. Many prayed for me, but I will never forget my middle son

Mark, a minister, striding into my cubicle, holding my wrist, and praying with authority. "Lord God, this is our mom lying here helpless. You need her and so do her children! Her single adults need her. She has unfinished work to do here on this earth. So raise her up, Lord! Strengthen her and give her back to all of us. I pray this in your strong, powerful name with the assurance that you will do it!"

I felt a bolt of energy enter my body, and I began to heal and regain strength. This is the way I want to petition the Big Physician on behalf of my patients!

God honors praying hearts. Often I tell patients, "The simplest, most powerful prayer you can offer is the word, *Jesus!* You may not have strength to say what is in your heart, but the Holy Spirit knows what's there, and you only have to call out *Jesus!*" Over and over in the New Testament, those in great need of healing called out, "Jesus, Son of David! Master!" And Jesus answered, "What do you want me to do for you?"

Dr. Benjamin Carson, the preeminent pediatric neurosurgeon, was the leader of the twenty-doctor team that performed twenty-eight hours of intense surgery in South Africa to separate Siamese twins joined at the back of their tiny heads. He speaks often of what a "God-sized job" the Lord did for him and the team of surgeons. "That was not me. I will admit that I have significant skills. But my skills are not that great. That was God!"

As the surgery proceeded, each blood vessel of the twins had to be identified and severed. "We had to decide which child would receive each blood vessel. As we struggled to separate the mass of abnormal blood vessels, I knew the Lord had to take over. Going through those blood vessels, I was taking a scalpel and cutting between very thin walls one or two layers thick. They were very fragile vessels that would have bled like crazy if you nicked them. I made those precision cuts for hours and hours and hours. It was almost like I wasn't there. It was almost like I was watching me. We only used four units of blood. With the other twins in 1987 it was sixty."

As the twenty-eight hours of intense surgery came to a close with the successful separation of the eleven-month-old babies, the "Hallelujah Chorus" poured through the loudspeakers as if on cue, and filled the air with the voices of angels. At the end of the surgery, one of the twins popped his eyes open and tried to pull his tube out. By the time they got to the Intensive Care Unit, the other was doing the same. Two weeks later, the twins were eating. By the end of two weeks, they were both crawling. So far there has been no evidence of any neurological impairment, a first for this type of operation.

"I pray before each operation for wisdom and guidance," says Dr. Carson. "I pray for God's direct intervention should it become necessary. There is a role for God to intervene when it comes to skill. It doesn't occur to you until you have reached your limit."

We caregivers need to get on our knees before God and renew our vision of the Living Lord and of ourselves as his representatives walking the corridors of hospitals, entering rooms, and asking, "How can I help you?"

Prayer

> *"Bear one another's burdens..."*
> *(Galatians 6:2)*

Healer of My Life,
Tears flowed as I left the hospital after dusk, and I could hardly see my way home. Tears of joy! To think that someone prayed for me! Someone who was vulnerable and transparent in his own grief set aside that grief to pray for me when he sensed I was in need of prayer also. Lord Jesus, he was right. There are so many germs of discouragement and defeat floating around. We need your protection. Bless him

forever, and bless you, Heavenly Father, for whispering my need to him. Give him the undisturbed sleep of a little child who has crawled up into your arms, Abba Father.

For Further Reading

Cousins, Norman. *Anatomy of an Illness as Perceived by the Patient.* Bantam Doubleday Dell, 1991.

Rupp, Joyce. *Praying Our Goodbyes.* Ivy Books, 1992.

Smedes, Lewis B. *How Can It Be All Right When Everything Is All Wrong?* Harold Shaw Publishers, 1999.

Wolff, Pierre. *May I Hate God?* Paulist Press, 1983.

Worden, J. William. *Grief Counseling and Grief Therapy: A Handbook for the Mental Health Practitioner.* Springer Pub. Co., 1991.